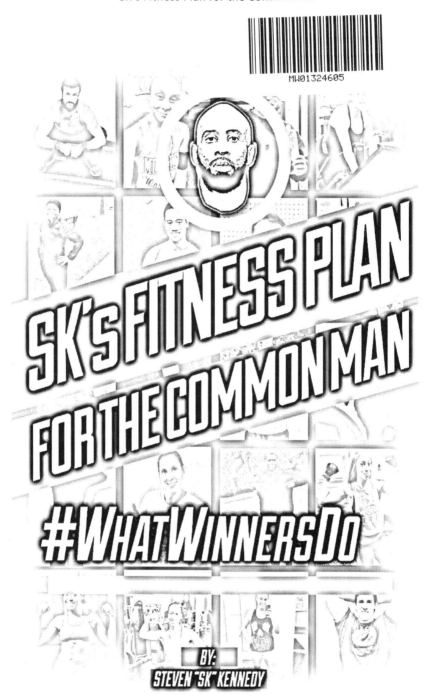

SK's Fitness Plan for the Common Man

Copyright © 2015 Mr. WhatWinnersDo

All rights reserved.

ISBN: 0692501339
ISBN-13: 978-0692501337

*Connie,
My favorite conservative jerk. Thanks for being a friend & giving me your support!*

SK

DEDICATION

This book is dedicated to anybody who ever had a dream, had the belief that dream could become reality, and then had the audacity to go after it.

SK's Fitness Plan for the Common Man

SK's Fitness Plan for the Common Man

To Inspire

To Inform

To Entertain

SK's Fitness Plan for the Common Man

LETS GO

SK's Fitness Plan for the Common Man

INTRODUCTION

#WhatWinnersDo

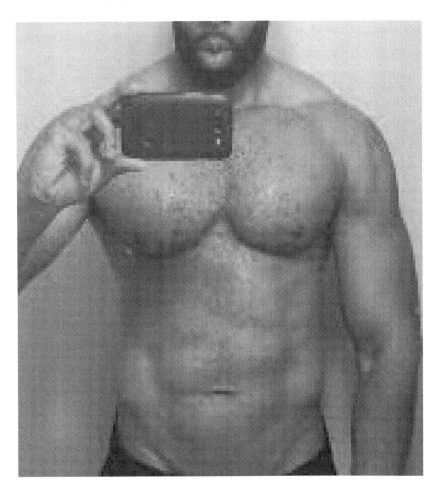

That's me, SK. A regular, common dude in his bathroom mirror taking regular, everyday selfies. I look pretty good, if I do say so myself (patting myself on back). Yes, hard work definitely pays off. This was not always my physique though. Let me give you some insight as to how I did it.

"SK, you fat as *hell* and out of shape." Those words, told to me by one of my best friends, Jeremiah, during a classic joking session, really struck a nerve. I went home that next night and took a long, real look at myself. I normally looked at myself in my bathroom mirror after a workout and would see a lie. I say a lie because I was looking at myself based on the weightlifting I had done and not what the lifestyle I was living had produced. My diet was horrid. I ate fried foods, cakes, ice cream, and pastas at any given hour of the day. I'm talking absolutely no chill. My cardio regiment was basically nonexistent. I mean one MAYBE two sessions of ten minutes on a low-speed Stairmaster™ machine a week. At that moment, I was able to see myself for what I had become, a *Bad Body* (term use to describe someone with an extremely out-of-shape figure). Don't get me wrong, I have never been a chiseled physical specimen in my life. In fact, the vast majority of my life, I have been known as "Big Steve," a husky, big intimidating dude. But what I saw at that moment disgusted me. I didn't even look remotely athletic anymore!

Embarrassed at what I had become, I vowed to myself that I would take steps to change this immediately. I had no idea how far I would or could go. But, I knew a change had to come. I was six foot one and 265 pounds that day, which was 35 pounds over my college football playing weight. Through a process that roughly took a year and a half, I was able to work my way down from 265 pounds with 23 percent body fat to 195 pounds with 11 percent body fat. The 195-pound mark being the smallest I had been since tenth grade in high school, some eighteen years ago. Pretty amazing transformation I must admit.

The most common question asked, after telling me how sexy or good I look, is how? How did SK go from a chubby goon-like guy who wears 3XL shirts and a 40-inch waist to a sleek, sexy adult medium shirt, with a 34-inch waist? How did SK go from being a bad body to having six-pack abs?

"Did you have surgery?"

"Are you sick?"

"Are you taking HGH?"

"Are you SK's younger brother?" (Cue Aloe Blacc's "The Man," as I put on my Beats By Dre™ headphones).

No, SK did not do any of that. The simple answer is that I simply worked hard. But, the truth of the matter is that it's so much more that went into it than just that. Working hard alone was not going to get me there. As my coach from college would often tell us, "Don't mistake activity for achievement." To be successful, I was going to have to work hard, be determined, and educate myself with information that would help me *flourish* on an epic level. It was a continuous process of seeking knowledge from as many knowledgeable people as possible, while paying attention to what did and didn't work for me.

Now, you could go online or to your local bookstore and find a million books on physical fitness, gym life, dieting, and so on. Most of those books will be 300-400 pages of in-depth information with a lot of scientific explanations and fitness jargon that is hard for the common person to follow. Let's face it, if you are a doctor, banker, lawyer, stay-at-home mom, engineer, hair dresser, or store manager working eight to ten hours daily, you probably do not have the desire to devote the time and energy that it would take to study and learn the information from one of those books of that caliber. The design of this book is to give you, the non-fitness guru, a few workable tips and tweaks that you can use in your everyday life to help you obtain your fitness goals. Each tip will contain an easy-to-follow explanation, preceded by a motivational quote that will also have an explanation. Because finding the motivation to consistently get you through the daily grind is just as important as your workouts and lifestyle changes. I can assure you that everything written here is what I personally practice, I can attest to its effectiveness, and I believe in it 100 percent. I have been blessed to work with and be advised by individuals who are well known and respected in the fitness world, and I just want to pass on to you the knowledge that was given to me because that's #WhatWinnersDo!

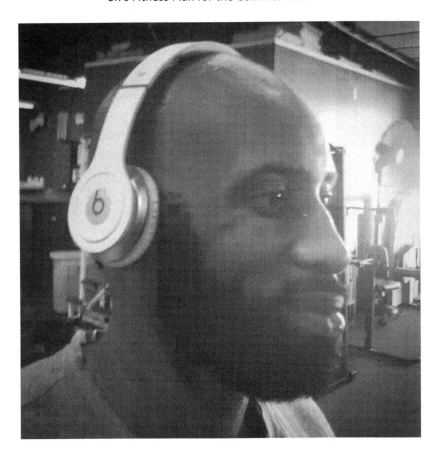

"Did you have surgery?"
"Are you sick?"
"Are you taking HGH?"
(cue Aloe Blacc's "The Man" theme music)

#WhatWinnersDo

CHAPTER 1

"Go flourish.

That's what winners do."

SK

These words have become my motto in life. It is a phrase that I use often to encourage friends and family for any situation. Although it is always well received, many admit to not fully understanding exactly what I mean.

We live in the world where most of us are basically trying to survive day to day. For the most part, we want to be able to pay our bills, eat a decent meal, get an alcoholic drink or two, catch a weekend movie, and just live out our lives. And people are good with that. But what I want you to know is that you do not have to work hard for that level of existence. That is the bare minimum, and God or the universe will always provide this for you.

What I want you to do is look past that. Achieve something out of the ordinary, defy the odds, test your limits, aim to be great, and flourish constantly. **To flourish is to achieve greatness, and greatness is not a single act, but a string of single acts that may manifest themselves in the appearance of a single act.** Therefore, we can say that flourishing is a lifestyle. And if you want to be a winner, then that is how you should aim to live because that is #WhatWinnersDo.

Wanna look good in clothes? Lose weight.

Wanna look good naked? WORK OUT.

First things first. Let's establish exactly what our mission is here. What exactly is it that *you* (yes you who just read that line) want to accomplish? It's pretty standard to hear someone on a daily basis say, "I want to lose weight," "I need to lose weight," or "I got to get this weight off me." Now, if that is your only goal, then that's a simple fix. Losing weight is nothing more than calorie counting. Everything you eat has a numeric calorie value. Every movement you do burns a certain amount of calories. Therefore, if you JUST want to lose weight, then you simply need to burn more calories in a day than you take in or eat. Repeat this daily, and sure enough you'll lose weight (shoulder shrug). It's that simple. You will notice your clothes fit looser, and you will look a bit better in them…BUT, when you take them off…well, that's another story. Let's just say you probably are not going to knock anyone's socks off.

I have a close friend who was constantly bragging to me about how much weight he was losing by calorie counting and not working out. "All I do is just calculate my calories. Man, I've lost 18 pounds!" Sounds good, right? Until one day we were at a pool, and it came time to take shirts off. This friend, who was once a stud athlete, now had the body of a regular Joe. What's wrong with looking like a regular Joe you ask? I guess the answer to that depends on your point of view and what you value. But, I once heard a very wise man say, "I just can't believe God put us here to be average," and it's that mindset that I share. You should want your body to look great! The best that it can! Do not get me wrong, losing bad weight is a good thing, but NOT the best thing by itself. But, when you combine it with working out, you now have the best of both worlds. That is why it is so very important to work out. Think of it like icing and cake. Losing weight is the icing, while working out is the cake. Icing is sweet and great for outer appearance and wearing clothes. But most of your substance is in the cake, which is below the icing and underneath your clothes. Now, if you get great cake and great icing, then you are winning (Kobe Bryant fist pump)!

You must understand that when I say *work out*, I'm not talking about using temporary measures to expedite your weight loss or reach a short-term goal. I'm telling you that **you should add working out into your lifestyle permanently.** There are so many advantages and benefits to doing so. Working out directly contributes to improving a wide range of aspects in your life.

Emotionally

Generally, people who work out are more stable emotionally and have better moods. Working out allows you to release stress and pent-up frustration and energy. Also, it gives you a sense of accomplishment, which makes you feel better overall about yourself.

Mentally

Working out effects the brain in a manner that can strengthen your memory, mental sharpness, and ability to focus for longer periods of time.

Physical health

Let's state the obvious. Working out makes a person's body stronger, which helps the body function better. People who work out live longer and have fewer health issues. Ladies may be surprised to learn that working out can help control or reduce symptoms associated with their menstrual cycle. Men may be surprised to learn that working out can drastically increase a man's sexual performance. Go ahead and get him that gym membership, ladies!

Appearance

Last, BUT DAMN SURE NOT LEAST, working out improves your appearance. Let's be real. Fellas, you want to be able to take your shirt off at the beach, and watch the ladies stare. You want your girl to stare at you the same way she stares at that hot dude she likes on TV like Idris Elba, Brad Pitt, Hugh Jackman, and so on. Ladies, you want to put on your hot short dress, and have all the guys trying to *holla* at you in the club. You want to walk the hot beach sand in your sexy bikini. You want to see that lustful fire in your man's eyes when he looks at you getting dressed. You want to wake up every morning, go to your bathroom mirror and say, "Mirror, mirror on the wall……DAMN I LOOK GOOD!!" And that is why you must work out because doing so will make all those things possible.

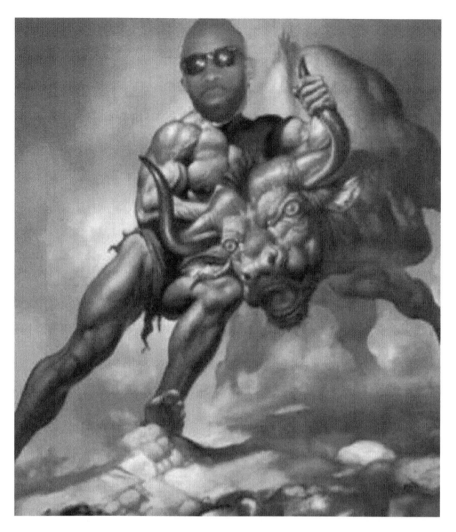

That's SK, in an epic battle (which really happened), literally taking the bull by the horns. And like me, you should take that same approach when it comes to your health and appearance by working out!!!!...Man I'm *swole*!

CHAPTER 2

"You can cheat on your boyfriend or girlfriend.

You can cheat on your job.

But don't cheat your body.

Because you can get another boyfriend or girlfriend.

You can get another job.

But you only get one body."

DAN AUSTIN

The person who created this quote is one of the strongest men in the world (Look him up). He called this the Weight Room Motto. Its meaning stresses the fact that in many aspects of life, we get do-overs, redos, makeups, or second chances at doing things. If you get fired from your job because they caught you sleeping, then you could make sure to always be awake and alert at your next one (or not get caught, LOL). If your girlfriend or boyfriend breaks up with you because they caught you being unfaithful, then the next time around, you could make sure to be faithful to that person (or again, not get caught, LOL). But, with your body, there are no do-overs, redos, or second chances. The things you do to your body now -- bad dieting, not working out, using abusive substances like drugs and alcohol -- all carry an accumulative, continuous effect. Body parts and functions will not look or work how you want or need them to later because of what you do now. It's like having a brand new car and driving it with reckless abandonment for years. It will end up breaking down on you long before it's supposed to. Everyone will age and all of our bodies will eventually fail us. BUT, we can play a huge roll in how that process goes. So stay faithful to yourself and never cheat your body. That's #WhatWinnersDo.

Free-weight back squats

LEARN 'EM

DO 'EM

LOVE 'EM!!

Without a doubt, **the most effective weightlifting exercise you can do is free-weight back squats.** I'm sorry fellas, it's not bench press. **No exercise is more effective for burning calories and fat.** If you were stranded in a gym and were told you could do only one exercise for the rest of your life, (yes, I know that would be ridiculous, but play along) your best option would be free-weight back squats.

For starters, free-weight back squats primarily work the quad, hamstring, and butt muscles. These are three of the largest muscles in the human body. The larger the muscle, the more energy it takes to work that muscle; thus, the more calories and fat you burn. Let's look at this concept logically. Your index finger is controlled by muscles, right? Flex and bend that finger fifty times. You were probably able to do this without any stress (if not, man you might be in trouble, LOL). Now, stand up and try to do fifty air squats (squats with only your body weight). You probably made it somewhere between twenty to thirty before the burn you felt in your legs made you stop. You may even be a bit out of breath. This just goes to show the difference between working smaller verses larger muscles.

Now you will hear people say that they prefer to do leg presses over free-weight back squats. They will have you to believe that the leg press is just as effective as squats. (Charlie Murphy voice)

WRONG!!! While leg press is an effect exercise, it's nowhere near as effective as free weight back squats. You may know someone who can get on a leg press machine and push 800 pounds, but struggle with 185 pounds doing free-weight back squats. This is because of the additional secondary muscles required to do free-weight back squats. You may have noticed and become annoyed that I keep referring to them as *free-weight back* squats. AH HA!!! There's a reason to the madness. When you use free weights, as opposed to machine weights, you must use your stabilizer muscles. These muscles, which include your core or abdomen, are responsible for maintaining balance, while the other muscles move the *free weight*. In addition to your stabilizer muscles, the shoulders, calves, and back are also engaged during this exercise. REMEMBER, the more muscles that you use equates to more fat and calories being burned.

A free-weighted back squat, while extremely effective, is not really a natural movement. For that reason, if you aren't experienced with doing them, you may want to seek the help of a trainer or someone experienced to help you learn the proper form and movement. I've trained many people to do them, and at first they all struggle with the awkwardness of the movement. Just be patience and persistent. I promise you the results will be worth it.

SIDEBAR The deeper you are able to go, the better the benefits. There is a theory that going deep in your squats is bad for your knees. Wrong! As long as you keep proper form and keep your weight disturbed from the balls of your feet to your heels (never on your toes), there is minimal, to no stress on your knees. The key is your hip flexibility. If you have tight hips, they will hamper your ability to go low without moving the weight from your heels and glutes to your knees and quads. The solution to this is to stretch your hips daily to loosen them up. Run an internet search for *hip stretches* and an array of different exercises will come up. Using any of them on a daily basis should allow you to notice a difference in a week or two. Now, go flourish.

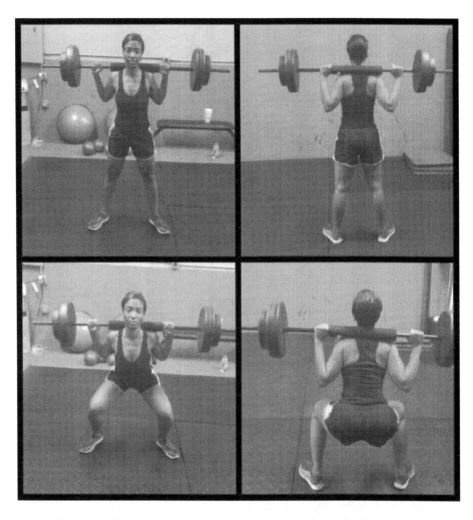

Your feet should be a little further than shoulder-width apart and should be positioned naturally on the ground.
The weighted bar should rest on your shoulders.
As you squat, keep your back straight and face forward, do not look down or up.
Use your glutes and hamstrings to lift yourself up to standing position.

REPEAT

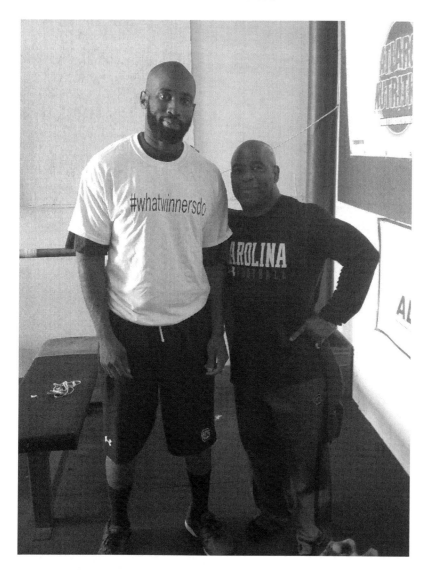

There he is standing with SK! The man, the myth, the legend, Dan Austin!!! He's been the head strength coach at five different collegiate universities. He's trained over a hundred professional athletes. He's a nine-time, world power lifting champion; sixteen-time national power lifting champion; and a member of the Power Lifting Hall of Fame. This guy definitely knows his stuff, and he is SK's go-to source for all fitness and training questions.

CHAPTER 3

"There are two types of pain in life. There is the

pain of discipline and the pain of disappointment. If you can

handle the pain of discipline, then you'll never have to deal

with the pain of disappointment."

Nick Saban

I got this quote from Nick Saban, who is currently the head football coach at the University of Alabama and universally regarded as one of the greatest college football coaches of all time. He is known, throughout the football world, as a coach who works his team extremely hard and demands discipline during their preparation. Consequently, year in and year out, his University of Alabama teams are regarded as the best in college football.

If you want your body to flourish on an epic level, that's the kind of attitude that is required. Trust me, it is not going to be easy! Being disciplined is one of the hardest things to do in life. It is what generally separates regular achievement from greatness. There are going to be times when you do not feel like going to the gym. So many times I woke up, body aching, and dreading my workouts. There will be days that you want to eat foods that are not in your current diet. I cannot tell you how many times I lay in bed in what felt like physical pain, fighting off the urge to eat some doughnuts or cookies. It is going to be tough, my friend.

Now, people around you will pacify you with statements like, "It's okay, everyone deserves a cheat day," or "missing a day of working out here and there won't hurt," to make you feel alright about giving in. That's what an average person does. But if you can stay disciplined and keep your eye on your goal, months from now, you will not have to live with the pain of disappointment.

"I wish I would've worked out everyday like I was supposed too."
"I wish I would've stayed on my diet the entire time."
"I wonder how much better I would be if I would've stayed disciplined?"

That pain is far greater and longer lasting than the pain it takes to be disciplined. That pain can and will eat at you forever. Whereas, the pain of discipline is temporary.

So pick a goal and a strategy on how you will get there. And stay disciplined until you reach that point. That's #WhatWinnersDo.

Want to work on your abs?

PLANK!

Planks are by far, without a doubt, the most effective exercise to work your abs and core. Every time I work with Willis Ham, AKA, the Ab Technician, we do a regiment of plank exercises to fire up our core. Now, I know you do 300 crunches every night before you go to bed, but they are not as effective as you believe. Matter of fact, you are kind of wasting your life doing crunches. Let me explain.

Your muscles are all responsible for a certain movement. To grow or work a muscle, you must put resistance against its intended motion or purpose. For example, your bicep is responsible for pulling your forearm towards your face. If you want to work it, then you need to put resistance against that movement (a weighted curl). The main function of your core, which is a group of muscles that include your abdominals (abs) along with some back, hip, and butt muscles, is to (believe it or not) keep your body upright. I know you're probably looking confused right now. But if not for your core, gravity would pull your body over. When you plank, you are isolating your core against the pull of gravity. This constant muscle tension is the best isolated work you can do. It will give you the tightness around your stomach area that you desire.

Crunches or sit ups are basically squeezing your abs together and up. This is indeed work, but nowhere near as effective. **Matter of fact, unless you can hold a plank for one minute, there is really no reason for you to do crunches.** Not to mention, you can change your position and work every section of your abs. A traditional plank works the front wall of your abs most. If you want to put more stress on your obliques, then take turns planking on each side. For your lower abs, you can lie on your back, and hold your legs up six inches off the ground. You can create a routine where you do each position for forty-five seconds, consecutively. Playing with routines like this will give you a really effective burn.

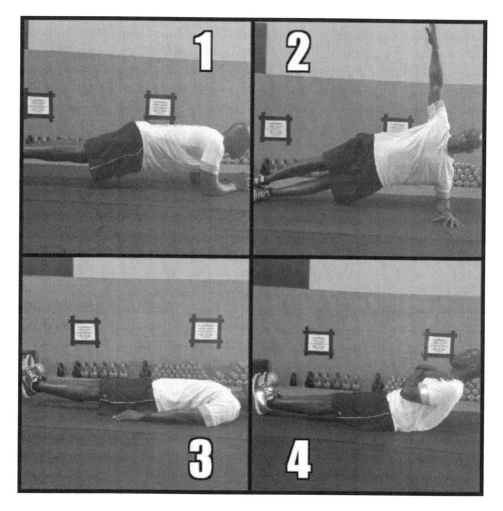

There are multiple ways to do your planks:
1. A standard plank works the entire abdominal wall.
2. A side plank (alternating sides) puts more stress on your oblique muscles.
3. A six-inch plank stresses the lower abdominal area.
4. A forty-five-degree lean stresses the top abdominal area.
Proper technique is paramount. So, consult with a trainer to be sure you are doing them properly

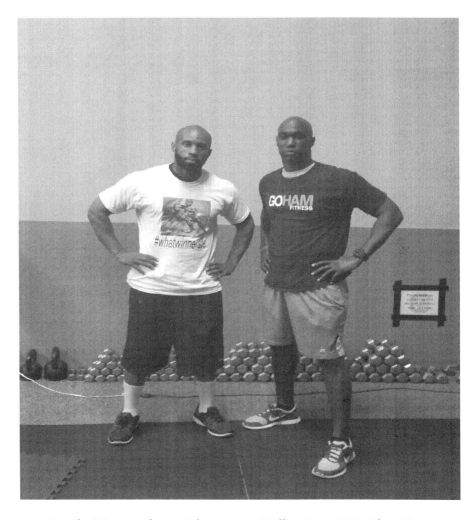

Here's SK posted up with my guy, Willis Ham, AKA, The AB Technician at Go Ham Fitness. Best abdominal and core trainer east of the Mississippi River (#honestdialogue). He's definitely a big reason why SK's abs are flourishing on an epic level!

#WhatWinnersDo

CHAPTER 4

> "Whether you think you can or whether you think you can't, you're right."
>
> Henry Ford

I honestly do not believe people understand the power of the mind. Some of the most amazing feats ever accomplished in the world happened simply because a person believed they could do it. I meet people all the time who come to me and say, "SK, I wish I could get in good shape….But I can't." My retort to them is always, "You're right." That always gets a crazy look from them. In their mind, they are saying, "WOW, why did he crush me like that?"

Look, no matter what I or anyone else says you can do, it does not matter if you don't believe it yourself. You must understand that you can do whatever you want, if you will simply start by believing in yourself. Positive thoughts and speaking things into existence is a real phenomenon. If you continuously think positive thoughts and speak positive words, eventually those things will begin to manifest themselves in the universe and in your actions. REMEMBER, do not defeat yourself before you even begin. Believe in your ability to change your body and flourish, and it will happen for you. That's #WhatWinnersDo.

Want to burn more calories and fat?

SPEED UP YOUR WORKOUTS!

People step to me in the gym all the time and say, "SK, I'm working out x days a week. But I'm not seeing the results I want. What do I do?" My first response is always, "You need to burn more calories and fat." To which they reply, "Well, how do I do that?" My simple answer, "Speed up your workouts."

Workout pace and time is everything when you are in the gym with the goal of burning fat and calories. It does not matter if I'm working out with Dan Austin, or with Rock and Jack in The Steel Mill in Atlanta GA, fast tempo is always preached. NOW, I know the gym culture. OH YEAH, I know how you do! You do an exercise; walk to the water fountain; stop and have a quick conversation with a gym buddy; look at your phone; check your Facebook®, Twitter, and Instagram™; take a workout selfie (Okay, I'm definitely guilty of that one!); walk back over to do another set of your exercise; and then repeat that process all over again. This is common for most people, and while they are getting the work done, they are not getting the full potential benefit from their workout.

Most people believe, when it comes to burning fat, it's about sweating a lot. But this is not necessarily true. Sweating is your body's way of controlling its temperature. If it's hot during your workout and you sweat a lot, does that mean you burned more fat than when you did the same workout when it was cold? No. Does a swimmer burn a lot of calories? Yes. The key thing to know, as my guy Ken Taylor pointed out to me, is that burning fat is directly related to your heart rate. The number to target is 120 beats per minute (bpm). When your heart rate is below that target number, you are burning your body's top layer fat. This is basically like fat around your arms, neck, and legs. This is what you typically burn during a slow-pace workout, while walking on the treadmill, using the elliptical machine, and so on. Once you get your heart rate to 120 bpm, your body begins to burn major, deep fat that is mainly in your mid section area and stomach, which is what most people desire. This is typically what you would reach during a fast-pace jog, sprints, and high-intensity workouts. **The higher you get your heart rate up, the more fat you will burn in this process.**

To achieve this, you do not have to necessarily change your workout regiment. You only have to speed up your pace. Monitor and lessen the length of time you rest between exercises. Cut out trips to the water fountain and distracting conversations with gym buddies. Time your workouts. Then come back the following week, and try to improve on that time. Be competitive with yourself.

So let's address the obviously question: How can you measure your heart rate to make sure it's where you need it to be? If you have a Galaxy 5S smart phone, it comes with an app that will magically (I say magically because I do not understand how it works) display your heart rate, and keep track as you work out. There are other electronic devices you can purchase that will do the same. Some will even alert you if it drops below a particular number, which in this case is 120 bpm. I personally use my breathing to approximately gauge my heart rate. Heavy breathing directly relates to a higher heart rate. I work out at a pace that constantly has me out of breath. As long as I feel a bit winded, I know I am safely over the magic number of 120 bpm.

Now, it is definitely a challenge. You will tell a noticeable difference in how you tire quicker, once you speed things up. But, you have to push yourself. The results you want are worth the extra effort it is going to take. Also, it will cut down on the amount of time you are actually in the gym. I consciously sped up my workouts from being an hour and a half down to forty minutes doing the exact same routine. This freed up almost an hour of my time. If you have kids, a 9-to-5 job, or both, you can definitely appreciate that because that hour can be used to flourish in some other area of your life.

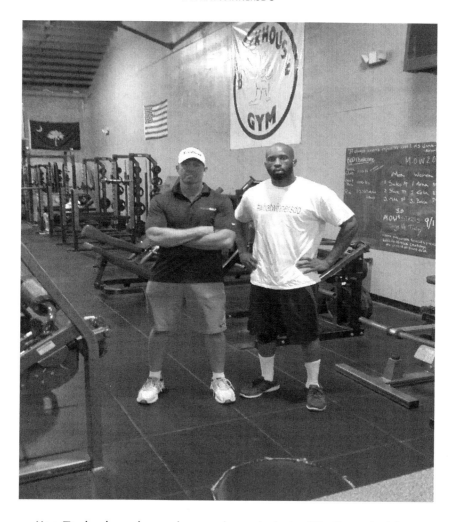

Ken Taylor has always been a huge help to SK. From holding multiple body building championships (Mr. South Carolina and Mr. Collegiate America) to owning his own gym to being a collegiate strength and conditioning coach, Ken is very knowledgeable in the area of sculpting a body. Throughout his career, he's trained with Arnold Schwarzenegger and a multitude of others. He is always available for solid advice and encouragement.

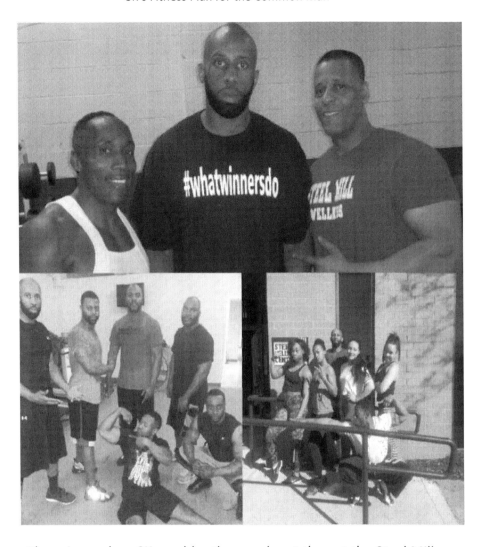

There is no place SK would rather work out than at the Steel Mill with the *Crew*. My guys Roc and Jack get the absolute best out of SK every time. "I GOT A SPOT FOR YA," is all you need to hear Roc say to know it is time to put in work. I have watched these guys transform many a body. If you are in the Atlanta, GA area, accept no substitutions.

#WhatWinnersDo

CHAPTER 5

> "In life,
>
> you either get better,
>
> or you get worse.
>
> Nothing remains the same."

Progression is an essential key to life in all aspects. Whether it is physically, mentally, socially, or financially, we should always strive to improve our current position. Too often, we become content with our situation and become complacent. The people around us will further this level of thinking. They will congratulate us and tell us that we have arrived. They will impregnate our mind with a sense that we have reached the mountain top, and there is nowhere further to go. But do not be fooled. We cannot maintain or hold on to the same position in life. There is no plateau on which to sit, once we have reached a certain point. Realize that if we are not building up, then we are sliding down. We are either growing or diminishing. Understand that there is always a higher level we can reach. There is always another mountain to be conquered, another river to be crossed, another pound of muscle to be gained, and another pound of fat to be lost. For you see, while perfection is an imaginary concept, we should always work and push towards it as if it is within our grasp. Continue to build and get better, that's #WhatWinnersDo.

Every month,
change your work out routine.

So let's say you have been on a workout regiment for two months. You have finally gotten to the point where you do not feel as if you are going to die after your workout. As a matter of fact, you feel as if you have conquered your workout and can pretty much breeze through the routine...TIME FOR A CHANGE!

Previously, I have expressed to you the importance of being consistent with your body to achieve maximum functionality. That principle does not apply to building and developing your muscles and burning fat. Let me explain.

When you work out, you are actually breaking down your muscles. To counter this, your body repairs the damaged muscle and builds it up a bit to withstand another incident like the one that just occurred. Confused? OK think of it like an earthquake hitting a city, and your body is the city. After the earthquake, the city rebuilds all the damage and makes the buildings stronger in case another earthquake hits. This way, the city will not be in as bad a shape the next time. Now, if the same earthquake happens again, the city will be a bit better prepared for it. This process is continuous until the city reaches a point where it is not phased by the earthquake. Your body treats your muscles the same way. After every workout, your body will repair your muscles based on what workout you did, in an effort to be better prepared in the event that it happens again.

The longer you continue to do the same workout, the fewer repairs your body will do on your muscles. Thus, you will begin to get diminishing returns on your workout and your body may eventually plateau, meaning your workout will stop giving you results. THAT AIN'T WHAT YOU WANT! Nobody wants to go to a gym and work out for an hour and not reap real benefits. To combat this, you will need to **change your workouts to create muscle confusion or as I like to say,** *shock the body.*

There are several ways we do this. You can work the same muscle, but use a different exercise. For example, if you are doing bench press for your chest, you may want to change and do dumbbell bench press instead. You can increase or decrease the repetitions (reps) you do relative to the increase or decrease in the weight you use. For example, if you are squatting 100 pounds for eight reps per set, you can change to 150 pounds for four reps per set. You could also drop down to 80 pounds for fifteen reps per set. Either of those changes could make a positive difference in your results.

This goes for cardio work as well. If you normally jog a mile, try running several series of sprints as a changeup. If the treadmill is your machine of choice, you may want to try the elliptical or Stairmaster™ machine.

My preferred method to shock the body is to do a completely different workout. Generally, I will find someone who I figure has a good workout routine and work out with them for a few days. People are generally ecstatic to have you work out with them, if for no other reason than to show off how great their workout is. "You're finally trying to step up to the big leagues?!" is the type of foolishness you will hear them say (SMH). You may even struggle a bit following their format. Do not become discouraged and question the level of your own workouts. This does not necessarily mean their workout is better than yours; but it more so represents the unfamiliarity your body has with this foreign regiment. "Yeah, we work out for real over here! None of that play-play stuff you do" (SMH and RME). If you can withstand this tomfoolery, then this can be a very effective tactic. Embrace the challenge, and know that your gains from doing so will only enhance your ability to flourish.

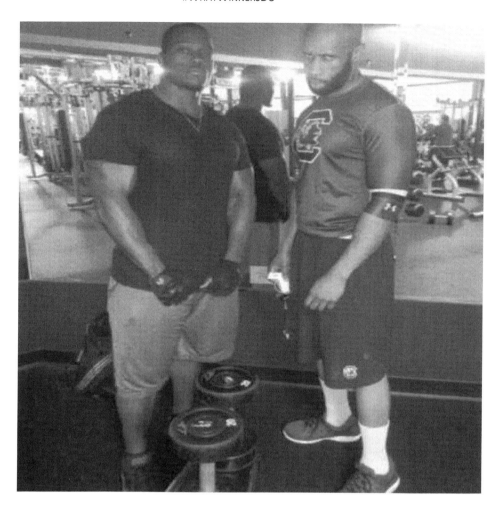

This is an old teammate of mine, GC (Gamecocks)!!!!! He is always willing to tell you about his great workouts. Guys like him are great for a change-of-pace workout. But, as you can see by my facial expression, I was not really impressed.

CHAPTER 6

"Do you not know that in a race all the runners run, but only

one gets the prize? Run in such a way as to get the prize."

> 1 Corinthians 9:24
> New International Version

"I returned, and saw under the sun, that the race is not given to

the swift, nor the battle to the strong, neither yet the bread to

the wise….but time and chance happen to them all."

> Ecclesiastes 9:11
> New International Version

I hold both of these biblical passages near and dear to my heart. They both express a principle that I strongly value. Everyone has an opportunity to win and succeed. In this life we live, the outcome is not predetermined. You do not have to spend your life out of shape or unhappy with your physical condition. You have the ability to change your body. You can win the race! You simply have to work in a way that will obtain the results you want. The runner who wins the race is not necessarily the faster or strongest. You may see people around you who are in better shape than you. They may get results quicker than you. Do not get discouraged! Everyone's body is different and grows and changes at its own pace. Focus on you! Focus on your race! Make sure that you maximize every workout. Each workout you do is the most important workout you have ever done because it is what you are doing at that moment. How do you run in a way to win the prize? Maximize the moment, be consistent over time, and have a great attitude while doing it. That's #WhatWinnersDo.

Cardio...

A necessary evil

Let's make this clear, SK does not like doing cardio. I never have, and I never will. You may feel the exact same way. But you will have to come to terms with the fact that if you want your body to truly flourish, you have to make it a part of your routine.

Cardiovascular exercise is basically any exercising you do that gets your heart rate up for an extended period of time. Remember, I stated earlier that if you want to burn more fat and calories during your workout, you should focus on getting your heart rate to 120 bpm or above. Cardiovascular exercises are an extension of that principle and the most effective way to get your heart rate above 120 bpm.

Now, when you start doing your cardio, realize that Rome was not built in a day. You will not be able to win a 5K race when you start. **Just like everything else in life, it takes time to get better and build up endurance. The key is to set goals for yourself, and figure out a systematic way of achieving them.**

For example, let's say you want to be able to run a ten-minute mile, nonstop on the treadmill. But, presently can only jog at a speed of 6 mph (equivalent to a ten-minute mile) for two minutes consecutively. You may start off on your first week (doing three cardio days per week), doing a ten-minute session alternating between walking at a speed of 3 mph and jogging at a speed of 6 mph every minute. That would give you five minutes of walking at 3 mph and five minutes of jogging at 6 mph. The second week, go to jogging at a speed of 6 mph for one and a half minutes, and alternate with a walking speed of 3 mph for one minute over a ten-minute period. This will give you six minutes of jogging, which is progress. The third week, start off jogging at 6 mph for two minutes and alternate to walking at 3 mph for forty seconds. That puts you at eight minutes of jogging for a ten-minute period. By the fourth week, you should be at the point where you can jog the entire ten minutes without breaking (FIST PUMP)! It is methods like this that will help you make adequate progress.

Week 1

| Walk 3 mph | 1 min |
| Jog 6 mph | 1 min |

Repeat for 10 consecutive minutes

Week 2

| Walk 3 mph | 1 min |
| Jog 6 mph | 1.5 min |

Repeat for 10 consecutive minutes

Week 3

| Jog 6 mph | 2 min |
| Walk 3 mph | 40 sec |

Repeat for 10 consecutive minutes

Week 4

| Jog 6 mph | 10 min |

The other important thing I want you to know about cardio is the wide variety of options available to you. You should not limit yourself to just one form of cardio, especially running or jogging. Running or jogging can cause extra wear and tear on your knees and feet, which could lead to injuries, arthritis, or both. Your local gym has some useful cardio machines like the elliptical, Stairmaster, stationary bikes, or cable rows that all can be used for effective cardio workouts. Swimming is also a great source of cardio. It gets your heart rate up, forces you to use all your muscles, and presents no wear and tear on your joints.

In addition, in your gym and throughout your city, there are many cardio exercise classes available for you to take. Zumba™ dance and Cycle Spinning™ are two hugely popular classes that are excellent sources of cardio exercises. These energetic group activities are filled with great music and commentary that push you past your limits, while *almost* making the cardio experience fun.

Whatever cardio exercises you choose to engage in, it is important to remember to constantly push yourself. Whether it be increasing your speed or distance, progression is a key element, if you want to burn as much fat as possible and flourish.

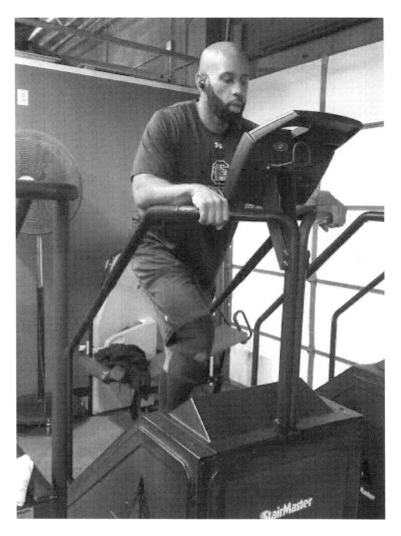

This machine is the absolute devil but, MAN, is it effective. Cardio is definitely one of the hardest things to do consistently, even for SK. But, if you want to flourish on an epic level, you must embrace it.

#WhatWinnersDo

CHAPTER 7

"You got to be comfortable with being uncomfortable."

Mike Tyson

This quote has been said by many a person, but I first encountered it while reading a Mike Tyson interview. He talked about how champions exist in a state of being constantly uncomfortable. They do this because being uncomfortable promotes growth, whether it be physical or mental.

Look, when you are working out, your body will eventually become uncomfortable. Phenomena such as being out of breathe, fatigued, and weakened will all occur. But, the truth is that these occurrences are necessary for you to grow and get the results you want. You have to learn how to embrace that aspect of the grind. Mike says that "anybody can do what they have to do, but the greatest people do it like they love it." Meaning they can mentally psych themselves into believing the pain is good. There are actually documentaries on people who are successful, on the highest levels, in sports and business that show that when these people are pushed to extreme limits, their brains react in a different way than normal people, in order to deal with the discomfort. They actually have trained themselves to flourish in situations of extreme discomfort. Instead of quitting or cowering back, they focus and push harder because they know this is when growth and success happens. They cannot wait to feel that shaking sensation during planks. They look forward to giving that speech in front of 5,000 people. They seek out that burning sensation when doing high repetitions while lifting weights. They cannot wait to make those cold calls every day. They love feeling out of breath, feeling almost to the point of choking, while jogging on the treadmill. They love pulling all nighters at work. That's what separates them.

So for you, who want those nice abs, chiseled chest, and firm booty, the next time you are working on that and you become uncomfortable, CELEBRATE and embrace that moment, knowing that feeling is going to get you the goals you desire. Push yourself to new limits. That's #WhatWinnersDo.

You have to learn the difference between being hurt
and being injured.

On your journey to a better you, which will consist of lifting weights, aerobic classes, cardio and other physical activities, you will probably experience, at one time or another, pain and discomfort in your body. Frankly, it comes with the territory. You see, working out forces your body to do things it's not accustomed to doing. So all that pushing, pulling, bending, and twisting you do is going to cause a lot of aches and pain. The problem is that once these events occur, many people stop immediately and completely discontinue working out. "Yeah SK, I used to work out. But, one day my foot started hurting. So I stopped." I let them know that was not their sign to throw in the towel.

Experiencing pain and hurt is definitely not necessarily a good thing but it's also not necessarily the worse thing. You have to learn the difference between feeling pain and being injured. **If you are hurt, then you are just experiencing discomfort/pain and can continue. But, if you are injured, it means something is structurally wrong with your body, and you need to stop.** It can be very tricky telling the difference and no one can tell you with 100% certainty what's going on with your body. Push yourself through the pain, but use your better judgment when something does not feel right. When in doubt, always err on the side of caution.

But, do not let aches and pain stop you from getting to your goal. When I hear people say they stopped working out because of an ache or pain, it saddens me (SMH) because there are plenty of other options. For one, you can lighten up the load. By reducing the amount you are doing, you can relieve stress in the hurting area. Another option is to simply do something different. If you feel pain doing squats, then maybe switch to doing leg curls or leg presses. And if it really bothers you, switch to doing some upper body so you are not using that muscle at all. Remember, anything you do is progress towards your goal.

Now if you believe something is seriously wrong, stop immediately and consider going to see a doctor. If you do not want to go to the doctor, then back off it a few days and give whatever is hurting you a chance to rest and heal. Applying a bag of ice to the affected area is also a good home remedy. It will help with pain, discomfort, and any swelling. DO NOT let one of these crazy trainers talk you into continuing doing something you know you can no longer do. They may mean well, but AGAIN it's your body, and nobody knows exactly what you feel but you.

I understand this segment may seem like a bit of a catch 22 situation. On one hand, I'm telling you to push harder through the pain. On the other hand, I'm telling you to fall back and take it easy. There's a fine line, and it's up to you to identify it for yourself. You just have to go hard and push through the pain; but listen to your body.

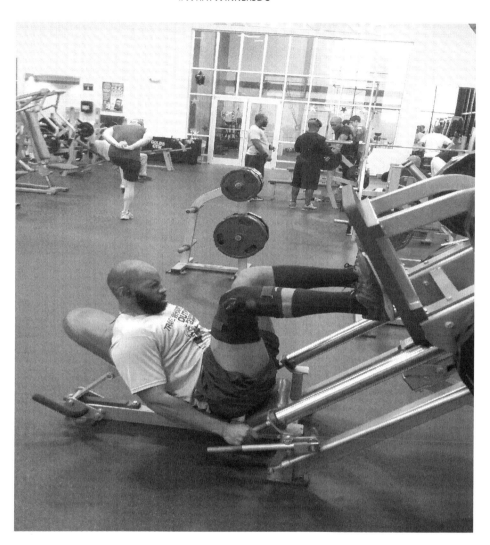

The pain on that face lets you know that 600-pound leg presses are no joke. But you know what they say in the gym, "No pains. No gains bro!!!"

CHAPTER 8

> "Don't be upset by the results you didn't get,
> from the work you didn't do,
> and the commitment you didn't keep."

I have a friend who calls me what seems to be every six months to complain about how she has not lost the weight she set for herself to lose. I asked what happened, and she proceeds to tell me how she does not work out consistently and cannot stick to her diet plan. Now, I presume she is reaching out to me to get sympathy. But all I can ever give her is tough love. I mean, how can you be upset about not getting something you did not do the work for? How can you be disappointed when you did not honor your own commitment to yourself? You have to put in the work and stay committed to your goal and plans. It's not easy being the flourisher of all flourishers. If it were easy, everyone would do it. You have got to do the work! You have got to stay committed! No one can do it for you. There is not a shortcut to get you there. Remember, the results you want are on the other side waiting for you. So GET TO WORK, STAY FOCUSED, AND GO MAKE IT HAPPEN!! Because that's #WhatWinnersDo.

What NOT to eat:

You gotta stay away

from the white stuff.

Once I decided to really focus on my diet, I needed to figure out what foods I needed to give up. I posed this question to my guy, The Great Dan Austin. "Give up all the white stuff," he insisted. That includes flour, sugar, pasta, white potatoes, white rice, white bread, grits, and dairy. These white foods are bad because they aid in storing fat and causing digestive problems. Flour, sugar, pasta, potatoes, rice, and bread all have a common trait. Consumption of them can cause a serious spike in your insulin levels. Insulin is released in the body to feed your muscles. The problem with having too much insulin released is that the excess is used by your body to feed your fat. Now, as you can imagine, it's hard to get rid of fat when you are constantly feeding the very fat you are trying to burn away.

White bread, white rice, white pasta, and flour are all man-made or processed foods. That means they are not naturally made. You won't find these items at your local farmer's market. This means that they are lacking in fiber and other nutrients. My guy, Ryan Sacko, has a saying, "**If it wasn't available to eat 500 years ago, stay away from it.**" These are what we consider bad carbohydrates (carbs). They contain a huge amount of calories per serving. Remember, losing weight is burning more calories than you consume. And guess what your body does with excess calories?...YEP, it turns into fat. (Fat Albert voice) HEY HEY HEY!!!

If you are using flour, that probably means you are frying food. Fried food is very bad! Cooking oil is the worst. It is extremely fattening and bad on your metabolism. After thirty years of age, seriously limiting the amount of fried foods you eat is the best thing you can do for your diet.

Sugar is produced naturally. But, in modern times, people consume entirely too much of it on a daily basis. Think about it. Soft drinks, condiments, chips, syrup, and sweets all contain massive amounts of sugar. A major problem with sugar is that it hurts the body's ability to maintain its blood sugar level. When levels are too high, excessive insulin is produced. When levels are too low, the muscles do not get the amount of insulin they need and cannot flourish.

Potatoes are not the worst thing in the world to eat. But, they do have a high impact on the body's sugar and insulin level. The biggest issue is that people tend to smother them with all sorts of terribly fattening toppings: bacon, cheese, sour cream, salt, and butter. These toppings turn a moderately healthy choice into a bad one quickly!

Milk and other dairy products are things you must give up, or you must greatly reduce your intake. Dairy products are very high in fat. In addition, dairy products are one of the hardest things for your body to digest, which in turn slows down your metabolism. Soooooooo not only is it high in fat, but it causes you to burn fat slower.

Don't get me wrong, nobody enjoys a Sunday, after-church dinner plate of fried chicken, macaroni and cheese, my Aunt Diane's rice dressing, cornbread, with collard greens soaked in grease more than good ole SK. A plate full of macadamia nut cookies (the best cookies ever in the world) or my Aunt Linda's world famous chewies and a glass of milk, can make the bad cloud go away on any day. But, if you want to truly flourish on an epic level, you'll need to greatly reduce your consumption of these things, just as I did.

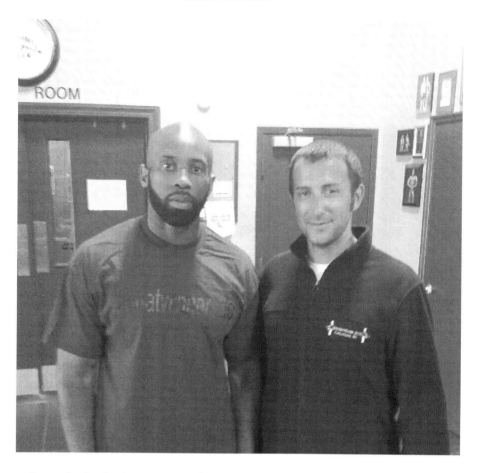

Ryan Sacko is the person who convinced me to get away from eating processed foods.

A former soccer captain at the College of Charleston, Ryan is a certified athletic trainer who has worked for the University of South Carolina as a trainer and a professor. He's also a workout warrior who is a master of creating alternative workouts. SK always gets great results working with him.

CHAPTER 9

> "Horses roam with horses.
>
> Cows graze with cows.
>
> They do not hang together."
>
> Farmer Joe

This passage, while indeed inspirational, is more so sound advice. As the story goes, Farmer Joe (local town farmer) knew a kid who was running around with a questionable crowd. He took the kid to the back of his farm, and they let all the horses and cows out the barn. "Look at them, kid. The horses are roaming with the other horses, and the cows are grazing with the other cows. They do not hang together. Now you need to figure out if you are a cow or a horse, and then go with your group." These words made the young man figure out that he was indeed hanging with the wrong crowd.

If your plan is to change your body, and improve your health, it would be very wise of you to associate with other people who are trying to do the same thing. There is real strength and benefit to having them around. It is great to have someone to encourage you during workouts. It is great to have an accountability partner to help you stay committed to gym days. Plus, the two of you can compare gym notes. In the Bible, Proverbs 27:17 says, "As iron sharpens iron, so does one friend sharpen another." Pay attention to the people around you. Make sure they are positive people who will help you stay focused and on task. In short, surround yourself with other winners because that's #WhatWinnersDo.

What TO eat:

Be a clean eating machine.

Now that I have killed your joy and told you what you cannot eat, it is only right that I let you know what you can eat. Most of the bad foods that we discussed have a good food counterpart. Now mind you, they may not be as appealing and tasty as the bad food choices. As a matter of fact, many of these healthy food choices may include a lot of foods you do not eat. Once you read some of the choices, you probably will immediately think to yourself, "I don't eat that." I know this because, at first, that was my mindset (LOL)! But, as my guy Derron Flood, the track workout specialist, told me, **"SK you can't want to have a Ferrari body and put 87 gas in it."** So I'd advise you to do as I did...SUCK IT UP.

I told you already that the white stuff is a no go. White bread, rice, and pasta are all bad! Now you may have interrupted that as me saying, "eliminate carbs from your diet." (ESPN's Lee Corso voice) NOT SO FAST MY FRIEND! I'm not telling you that at all. Don't get it confused. You need carbs in your diet. I'll repeat that. YOU NEED CARBS IN YOUR DIET. Carbs have a similar relationship with muscles, like mortar has with bricks. Carbs protect and hold your muscles together. A carb-deficient body is more susceptible to injury. Add to the fact that carbs supply energy to your body and mind. In other words, a carb-depleted body may not perform well during exercise, and you could not be as sharp mentally. Instead of eliminating all carbs, focus on eating good, quality carbs. Whole grain bread, rice, and pasta are great substitutions for their white counterparts. Whole-grain products are naturally made. So, they contain all the nutrients needed to be effective.

Now, I have bad news, and I have good news to give you. The bad news is that there really is no substitution for fried food. So you have to accept the fact that you are going to have to do without (extreme sad face). The good news is that you can still sauté your food. But instead of using vegetable cooking oil, you can use extra virgin olive oil (OK that wasn't exactly good news but still, LOL). Extra virgin olive oil is completely natural and contains lots of good fats (yes there are good fats) and other nutrients. Adding a little extra virgin olive oil to sauté your food, grease your pan, or to flavor your salad is definitely a good thing.

Sweet potatoes are a great substitute for white potatoes. Sweet potatoes contain less carbs, calories, and fat than white potatoes. You will be pleased to know that you can even get sweet potato French fries and sweet potato, potato chips as well.

Controversial

Sugar consumption is a major problem. Unfortunately, there is not a positive substitute. Brown sugar is nothing but regular sugar with color added to it (Yeah they fooled you). A key thing I did was to not drink as much sugar. Kool-Aid™, sodas, juices, lemonade, and so on are all loaded with absurd amounts of sugar. In a perfect world, you would just drink water 24/7. But, I refuse to drink water with my meals. (Coach Mike Singletary voice) CANT DO IT!! So, I started using artificial flavoring packages like Crystal Light®. These packages have no sugar in them, but give you a decent-tasting drink. This is where the controversy begins. You will have people who will debate with you that using the artificial flavoring is actually worse for you than drinking the beverage filled with sugar. Their reasoning is that since it is artificially made, the body does not know how to use it. This makes some sense, especially when you think about the quote Ryan Sacko gave me earlier, "If it wasn't around 500 years ago, its not good for you." BUT, this book is about what worked for SK, and I can tell you truly that I noticed a huge difference in my results, once I started drinking Crystal Light instead of soft drinks. My advice to you is to try it out, and pay attention to your body. See what type of effect substituting Crystal Light for beverages has on your body, and then you can decide whether to adopt it into your lifestyle or attempt something else. REMEMBER, everyone's body is different and may react differently to different things.

Dairy products are very high in fat and one of the hardest things for your body to digest. However, they are not particularly easy to substitute. My personal recommendation is to simply avoid using them as much as possible. But if you must, you may want to use almond or coconut milk instead of diary. Almond and coconut milk are both a lot less fattening than the dairy alternative. They are a perfect with for your cereal, and you can use them in any recipe that requires milk.

Choosing the right foods to incorporate into your diet will do several things for you: Boost your metabolism, improve your health, cause your body to store less fat, and generally make you feel good. The down side is that the healthy alternatives in this chapter may not be your first choice. REMEMBER, you are sacrificing today so you can flourish tomorrow. I know it sucks at the present moment. There were days when I wanted fried chicken soooooooooo bad. But, I held strong. And days, weeks, months later, when I saw the results I was getting, I understood at that moment that it was all worth it. And if you make that commitment, you will too.

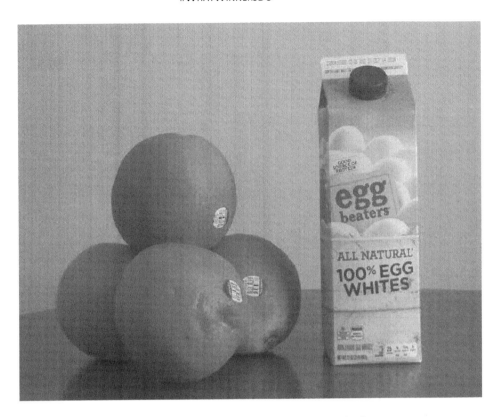

In addition to the food choices that I just discussed, these items are steady parts of my diet. Eggs whites are a great source of pure protein. I add them to basically any meal. Grapefruits, on the other hand, are great for burning fat. They are perfect for a between-meal snack. Adding these items to your diet will definitely pay dividends.

CHAPTER 10

> "When you take care of the little things,
> the big things take care of themselves."
>
> Lou Holtz

This is truly a profound statement made by one of the greatest college football coaches ever. I had the honor of playing for him and heard this nugget of wisdom time and time again. If you're overweight and want to get a six-pack stomach, it's not going to happen overnight, I promise you. To keep it real, it's not going to happen in a week, a month, or probably even a year! You see, that six pack is your *big thing*, and looking at the big thing can be overwhelming. But know that big things are made of lots and lots of little things. In this case, lifting weights, doing cardio, working your core, and following a proper diet are all the little things. If you look at yourself in the mirror, and let your mind wonder to think, "Mannnn I have a long way to go!" Then, it may begin to discourage you and kill your motivation.

"I can't do this."

"This is hopeless."

"This is too hard for me to do."

These are some of the more popular self-doubt statements people make in these situations. But, the key is NOT, I repeat, NOT to focus on the big picture. Focus on taking care of your little battles every single day, one day at a time. Eat what you're supposed to eat, lift weights when you planned to lift, and do the cardio you planned to do. "Win the day," is what people say. If you do this day in and day out, your *big thing* will take care of itself, and you will be where you want to be because that's #WhatWinnersDo.

WHEN to eat:

Eat your meals the

exact

same time every day.

Meal timing is extremely important for the simple fact that your mind and body don't talk. Think of it like a struggling married couple. The couple stays together day in and out, but they have poor communication. Although you may decide, in your mind, to wait an extra two hours to finish work before you eat dinner, this message is not received by your body. Self preservation is always your body's first instinct. So it panics and believes that you are literally starving. Once your body is in that mode, it begins to store and hold on to as much fat as possible. Reason being is that if you ever are really starving, the body burns fat to stay alive. So, when you do actually eat, instead of using all nutrients and digesting food, your body turns more of it to fat and stores it.

Why eat at the exact same time every day? Remember, your body operates best with regularity. **Eating at the exact same time will give your body a systematic comfort of function**. It will know exactly when to expect food and will use nutrients and digest waste fluidly knowing that it will be fed again at the next specific time. Your energy level will increase and not fluctuate from high to low, you will boost your metabolism, which will allow you to burn fat and calories steadily, and you may generally feel a lot better.

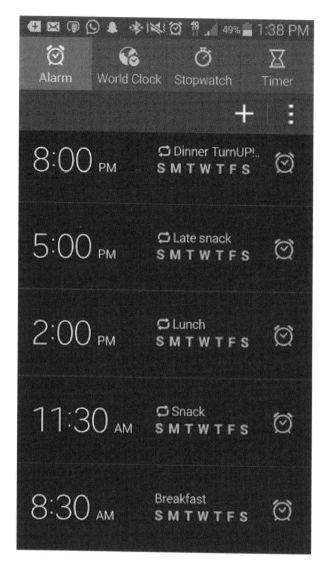

A busy schedule can easily make you forget about eating when you are supposed to. I mean, time can really fly by when you are focused on work or a task at hand. But thanks to these smart phones that 90% of us have, we can schedule our reminders!

CHAPTER 11

> "Don't stop believin'
> Hold on to that feelin'"
>
> Journey

At any given time, you can catch me singing this chorus. Definitely one of SK's favorite songs of all time.

Have you ever had that certain feeling when you are truly inspired? That feeling when you see a goal that you want to achieve, and you have an epiphany that it is indeed possible. Regardless of how far-fetched it may seem to others, you know you can do it, and you are determined to see it through. Take that same feeling where you realize that you will do whatever it takes to achieve the goal at hand, and hold on to it!

So often I see people in the gym, at the track, or on social media, and they are so full of newly found enthusiasm. You can see the fire in their eyes and hear the passion in their voices as they talk to you about what they are going to accomplish.

"SK, I'm going to get rid of this beer belly!"
"SK, I'm going to drop this weight and get back down to my college size!"

There's something about those encounters that literally sends a shiver down my spine. The sad thing is that if you find those people after a few weeks, they often have reverted back to their old ways and that fire, which was so amazing, has now died out. They lost it. They stopped believing in themselves and have given in to doubt. They believe the false reality that the goal they envisioned is too difficult, and they cannot accomplish it.

Do not fall victim to that frame of mind. Remember that spark you had when you first started. Keep that fire in your belly that keeps you going every day. Simply put, don't stop believing, and hold onto that feeling. That's #WhatWinnersDo.

Be a Mogwai.

Don't turn into a Gremlin.

If you are thirty years old or older, you probably remember the 80s hit movie, *Gremlins* (if not, I strongly suggest you look it up). In the movie, one of the rules was that you could not feed the Mogwais (small, cute, furry creatures) after midnight. When that happened, they morphed into evil green monsters (Gremlins). Well my friend, if you want to get in great shape, this is a strategy you should also use.

When you sleep, your body's metabolism and digestive system are all operating at its slowest points. Any food you eat late at night is digested extremely slowly, and what it does not digest, will be stored as fat. This means that the late-night, after-the-club trips to Waffle House®, Denny's®, and IHOP® must cease!

Now, there are some that will argue you down that there is no conclusive evidence that eating late contributes to weight gain. They basically say that "a calorie is a calorie" regardless of when you consume it. But, based on MY personally experience and research, I would have to disagree. I was a person who constantly ate late at night. Once I made a commitment to eat no later than 9:00 p.m., I started to notice a difference in my weight and morning energy level. REMEMBER, everyone's body is different. Stop eating late at night, and see what type of difference you notice. If doing this enhances your ability to flourish, then adopt it as a permanent practice.

SK's Fitness Plan for the Common Man

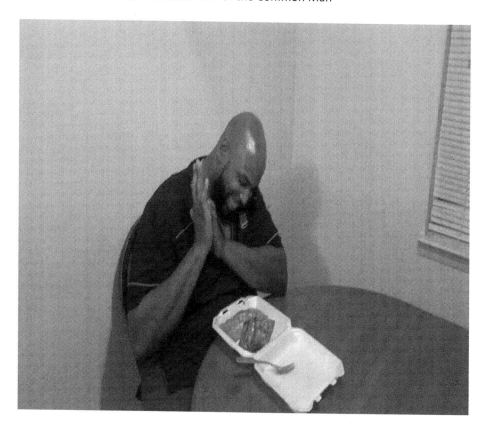

I understand that late night meal can be very tempting…………………………….

SK's Fitness Plan for the Common Man

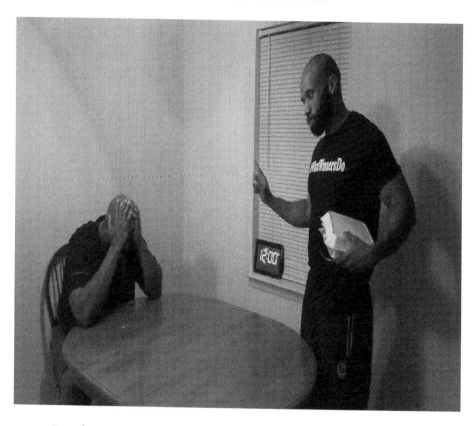

But if you want to flourish, you got to stay strong!!!!!!!

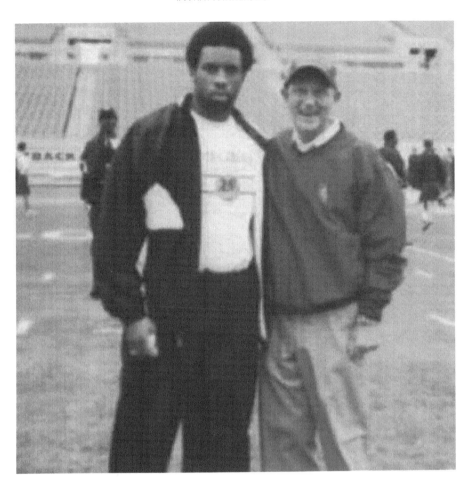

That's me, SK, standing with Lou Holtz, the legend himself. He is definitely one of the wisest and most inspiring people I have ever known. It was an absolute privilege to be able to learn from him for four years. Pay no attention to my haircut.

CHAPTER 12

Luke Skywalker: "OK, I'll give it a try."

Yoda: "No! Try not! Do! Or do not. There is no try."

Star Wars Episode V

This exchange in dialogue is taken from the movie, *Star Wars: The Empire Strikes Back.* In this scene, Yoda, the wise Jedi Master, is challenging Luke, his young Jedi apprentice, to perform a feat that, in Luke's mind, seems impossible. Luke, filled with doubt, attempts to casually tell Yoda that he will try. Yoda abruptly cuts him off and tells him, in his own special Yoda way, "No!" Do not try! Either do it, or do not do it! Trying is not an option. I hear this so much. Different people stating how they want to TRY to lose weight, TRY to get a six pack, TRY to eat right, TRY to get back in shape and so on. To use the word, TRY, indicates a lack of confidence, lack of commitment, or the presence of fear. People fail to understand that self doubt is the thing in life that will hinder you the most from flourishing. The human body and mind, together, can accomplish some truly amazing feats. The possibilities are endless. If you are going to obtain your goal, no matter how far away or far-fetched it seems, you have to become determined and confident in your abilities. Go at it with everything you have! Give it your absolute best effort! Know that it will happen! That's #WhatWinndersDo.

JUST SAY NO...

To fast food, buffets, and high-fructose corn syrup.

D.A.R.E to keep a kid off drugs! You remember that?! If you are near my age, 30s-40s, then you probably remember that program from elementary school that was designed to get kids to stay away from drug abuse. "JUST SAY NO!" was all they tried to drive into our heads. Well, I adopted that same motto for fast food, buffets, and high-fructose corn syrup, and you should too if you want to better your fitness level.

Fast food

Now when I say fast food, I'm talking pretty much ALL fast food chains. Regardless if they serve burgers, chicken, tacos, or pizza, they are all bad. Why you ask? Because the quality of food they serve is terrible. It's called fast food for a reason. They use poor grades of meat, lots of salt, lots of grease, and God only knows what else. There's always a report on the news about a restaurant, the type of meat they use, and the methods in which they store or cook it. There's even that documentary *Supersize Me* about a guy who ate McDonald's for an extended period of time and the effect it had on his body and health.

Now, I know what you're going to say, "SK, I go for the salads and fruit cups," or "Well I eat their egg muffins because they use real eggs." Let me ask you, if you were thirsty and the Devil (the guy with the horns and hoofs for legs) came to you and offered you a glass of water, would you take it? My thought is I do not trust anything that comes from an untrustworthy source. Even those salads are filled with an absurd amount of preservatives.

I understand fast food is extremely convenient and fairly cheap, but you are severely sacrificing quality, and **quality is what matters the most when dealing with your body**. I confess that one night, a few years ago, I decided to pick up a cheeseburger. MANNNNNN, I think I almost died after eating that thing. I literally had it coming up out of both ends that night. It took me about three days to feel right again. Now if you are eating this type of food daily, you can take this poison in with little to no problem because your body is use to it. But, clean up your diet for an extended period of time, and then try to eat one of those fast food burgers. Experience firsthand how awful you feel afterwards. You then can understand how counterproductive eating this type of food can be to your ability to flourish.

Buffets

Buffets and family-style meals (those feasts that you have at your grandma's house on Sunday) have three real issues: quality of food, quantity of food, and type of food. The quality of food they are serving is not top notch. I mean, think about it. Do you really think all-you-can-eat steak and lobster for $9.99 is going to be prime quality? Even at your grandma's house, look at the chicken. I'm sure there are a lot of legs and thighs being served. No coincidence that those are the two fattiest parts of a chicken. Remember, you want to put quality food in your body for it to perform optimally.

The next problem with buffets is that they encourage excessive eating. When you are trying to lose weight or improve your fitness, eating until you fall over is not a productive way to go about it. I mean, the caloric intake at those things is absurd. My suggestion is that they install a calorie ticker over everyone's table so you can look up and see the astronomically numbers you are taking in. Understand that when your digestive system is overloaded, it starts storing the excess food as, you guessed it, fat.

The last, but certainly not least, problem is the kind of foods people eat the most at buffets. It's a steady serving of white bread rolls, macaroni and cheese, rice and gravy, fried chicken, pork chops, pasta, cake, cookies, and sundaes (basically everything on the *what-not-to-eat* list). All the food you would find in the anti-flourish movement.

Now, do not get me wrong. On Christmas, Thanksgiving, Fourth of July and so on all bets are off, EVEN for SK! You can find me passed out on a couch, pants unbuttoned to give me room from being overstuffed just like anyone else. But on those special occasions, it's okay to let your hair down and indulge a bit. But if this is an every-other-day or even a weekly habit, like every Sunday after church, that's no bueno.

High-fructose corn syrup

This stuff is point blank bad for you. It's a cheaper, unnatural substitute for real sugar that is used in lots of grocery foods. I could go into a long scientific explanation about its negative effects but I will keep it simple and tell you that a steady diet of high-fructose corn syrup can contribute to diabetes, damage your immune system, speed up the aging process (make you look old), and it contains a dangerous poison, mercury. It has also been linked to causing obesity and weight gain. Safe to say, high-fructose corn syrup is bad stuff that will hurt your ability to flourish, and it is not #WhatWinnersDo. Stay away from this stuff at all cost. You can find it in your ketchup, syrup, potatoes chips, bread, barbeque sauce, soft drinks, juices, cereals, and a multitude of other items. You can basically find it in anything with added ingredients for taste. Look at the ingredients on whatever you buy. Pretty much everything you buy that has high-fructose corn syrup in it, has a natural sugar product right beside it. The natural sugar product may cost an extra dollar or two, but pay it! Trust me, it is worth it.

SK's Fitness Plan for the Common Man

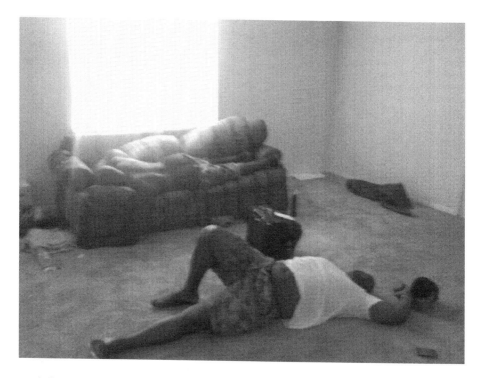

Did these guys just have a long night??? No, they are recuperating from a visit to the local Chinese buffet (Apparently they REALLY enjoyed themselves). Times like this are OK every blue moon, but definitely should not be a habit.

#WhatWinnersDo

CHAPTER 13

> "Some say the glass is half full.
>
> Some say the glass is half empty.
>
> But I ask you, what does it matter?
>
> JUST FILL IT UP!"
>
> — SK

Perspective is an important aspect of life. But too often, we dwell and focus too much on our current situation. If you are a pessimist, then people will say that you focus on how far you have to go. Pessimists usually speak about being discouraged because of their current situation and having to go so far to get to their goal. If you are an optimist, then people will say you focus on how far you have come. Optimists usually speak glowingly of their current situation, but lose some of their drive and become content with the success they have obtained. But my question to you is, in the grand scheme of things, what does it matter? Your current situation is only a starting point for the place you are today, based on what you did yesterday, and where you will not be tomorrow. Look, God put eyes in the front of our head and not in the back so we can focus on what lies ahead and not what is behind us. Keep your eyes and mind focused on the goals you are striving for. Stay hungry, and keep working hard because that's #WhatWinnersDo.

Drink a full glass of water

as soon as you wake up in the morning,

before each meal,

and before you go to bed at night.

Water intake and hydration are EXTREMELY important to being healthy and fit. As a matter of fact, outside of oxygen, nothing is more vital to your body's survival and function. While you could last about three weeks without food, you could only go about three days without water. To get your body into shape and work the way you want, you need to get it operating at its maximum functionality; meaning, all systems and parts are flourishing at their highest level. This will then make your body do things you want it to do, like digest food, burn fat, and develop muscle. Proper hydration is essential to ensuring this. And when I say proper hydration, I'm not talking about drinking Gatorade®, Powerade®, flavored water, or Diet Coke®. I'm talking about drinking regular H$_2$0, water! **There is no substitute for water.** The problem is, most people do not get nearly enough water into their body to have it reach that level of maximum functionality. Now, I am sure we have all seen the lady at work who carries a gallon jug of water with her and drinks it periodically throughout the day. I applaud the effort and commitment, but for you or SK, the everyday person, who really wants to carry a *big-ass* jug with them every single day?! Not SK! Using my method does two important things: It gives you the proper amount of daily water and it gives your body a steady, consistent schedule for water intake.

To reach maximum functionality, you need the proper amount and consistency. Remember, your body and mind DO NOT talk. So when you say, "I'll drink some water when I get off today." That memo is never relayed to your body, and it functions accordingly. Now let's break down the SK method.

The rule of thumb is that you take your body weight, divide it in half, and that's the amount of water in ounces your body minimally needs daily. You should be eating between four to six meals a day. A glass of 16 to 20 ounces of water before each meal (in addition to whatever soft drink you may drink with your meal), along with one glass at night and one in the morning, would put you somewhere between 96 to 160 ounces per day. Those numbers match up with a weight range of a person between roughly 190 to 320 pounds. You just have to adjust the amount of water to suit your body weight. But remember, the more water you drink, the better.

Drinking those glasses of water last thing at night and first thing in the morning are very important. The average person sleeps between six to ten hours a night. And since this is when you are in rest-and-recover mode, you definitely want to go to bed well hydrated so your body can work its magic properly. When you wake up in the morning, realize that you've gone six to ten hours without any water being given to your body. Most people wake up close to dehydrated. A full glass in the morning gives your body the juice it needs to pick up and operate again for the day.

Many people have the idea that drinking more water will cause their body to retain more water weight. While it makes logical sense that the more water you drink, the more water you have in your body, it is the opposite that actually happens. Once your body knows it is going to get a steady flow of water, it releases water weight easier because it knows that it gets water frequently. So it doesn't have to store as much water. It's kind of like when you are shopping and that shirt costs $100, but you have $110. If you know you are getting paid tomorrow, you will probably say "RING IT UP!" BUT, if you are not sure when the check is coming, you will probably want to chill and hold onto your $110 (LOL)!

Following the SK method will get you on your way to maximum functionality and proper hydration. Best way to gauge if you are indeed hydrated is by the color of your urine. A properly hydrated body produces close to clear urine (pee). You should be able to look at your pee and say, (Steve Urkel voice) "I AM CLEARLY HYDRATED!" BUT mind you, this does not include that sip of water you go get while you're bored at your desk, the water you drink to keep you hydrated during and after your workouts, or the bottle of water you drink in your office meeting to keep you from being too bored. Those are added bonuses or extra credit that your body will appreciate. The SK method just ensures that you get at least the minimum amount of water you need daily.

#WhatWinnersDo

GUESS WHAT......

#WhatWinnersDo

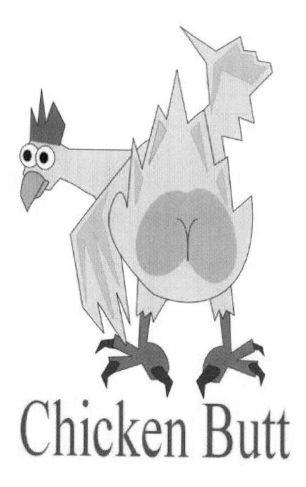

Chicken Butt

Okay, this has absolutely nothing to do with fitness and inspiration, but I love this joke.
(Yes, very childish I know)

LOL!!

#WhatWinnersDo

CHAPTER 14

> "If it's important to you, you will make time.
>
> If you can't make time, then it's just not that important to you."
>
> Lou Holtz

This is another gem I stole from good ole Coach Holtz. Everyone has a busy schedule. Life often bombards us with a multitude of tasks and obligations. "SK, I wanna get right, but I don't have the time." That is by far the common excuse I hear. "You can. But, you just choose not too," is what I always tell them. Hey, I understand you may be a single parent with two kids and a nine-to-five job, or you work a job that has you traveling city to city on a nightly basis, or you work a shift that does not allow you to get to the gym before it closes. But, there is always a way. It may require you to be creative and precise with your time and schedule. But, it is possible. You may have to get up an extra hour earlier to jog on your treadmill. You may have to download workouts onto your laptop to do in your hotel room. You may even have to work out on your lunch break. Doing those things and making those adjustments are not necessarily convenient. But, if it's important to you to improve yourself, you will make the time, and do them. That's #WhatWinnersDo.

Sleep the same time, same amount, EVERY DAY!!!

This part of the fitness plan may be a bit controversial. What I'm going to tell you more than likely doesn't match up with what your scholar trainer will tell you. But again, this entire book is devoted to things I have personally experienced and learned that work for me. Common belief is that you need eight hours of sleep nightly for your body to properly refresh. But it is my belief that your body can adjust to whatever amount of sleep you get as long as you do it on a consistence basis. Here's my personal reasoning.

There came a point in my life when I was working two jobs and still needed to work out. My day would go as follows:

7:00 a.m.   Wake up, get dressed, and head to the gym.
7:30 a.m.   Arrive at gym for a workout.
9:00 a.m.   Return home to cook breakfast, shower, eat, and get dressed for work.
9:45 a.m.   Leave for work.
10:00 a.m. Arrive at my office, and work until 3:00p.m.
3:00 p.m.   Change clothes, and head to my second job.
3:30 p.m.   Work my second job until 1:30a.m.
2:00 a.m.   Return home for the day. Fall asleep around 2:30a.m.
7:00 a.m.   WAKE UP AND REPEAT!

I was basically having twenty-hour days Monday through Friday and did this for a five-month period. Saturdays, since I was off, I would go do Bikram Yoga and then an hour of cardio. Sunday would be a lounge and relax day. That's a lot right? Yeah, I was doing the most. Now, based on the common rule of eight hours per night, my body should have been breaking down and falling apart. But, even to my surprise, during that time span, I was able to make sizeable gains in strength and muscle size. Friends and family who knew the schedule I was on, would always warn me.

"You're going to pass out."

"You're killing yourself."

"Are you crazy?"

But I never experienced an out-of-the ordinary problem. Remember, I have stressed that one of the important things your body needs is consistency. Once my body understood what the schedule was, it was able to adjust and adapt. Now, this is going to really knock your socks off. The entire time I was on this schedule, after the first week, never again did I have to use an alarm clock of any kind. YEP! You read that right. I went to bed around 2:30 a.m and woke up around 7:00 a.m every day all on my body's natural clock. THAT'S CRAZY RIGHT?! But when you have defined purpose and consistency, I assure you it can happen.

On one occasion, I was off and figured I'd get in a much-desired nap in the middle of the day. HUGE MISTAKE! I woke up feeling drained and felt a step off for the next few days. My pattern was broken, and my body didn't understand what was going on. Remember, your mind and body do not talk! Rest assured, that was the first and last nap I took during that time.

Now, am I telling you to only get four hours of sleep a night?

Absolutely not! I am just showing you what I was able to do as an example to dispel the notion that you have to have eight hours of sleep to refresh your body. Please know that there are additional ways to refresh and regenerate yourself. Doing things like yoga classes, swimming, sitting in a sauna, and massages are all great ways to keep your body fresh. Now remember, EVERYBODY'S body is different. You will have to figure out the amount of nightly sleep you need and what times work best for you. My biggest thing is that you be consistent to enhance your body's ability to flourish.

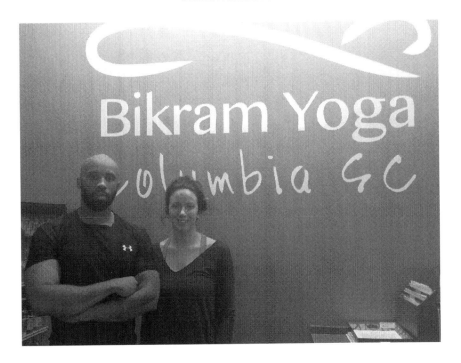

Hanging out with my buddy, Lacy, at Bikram Yoga Columbia, SC. Although SK is stiffer than a tree, taking these classes has been great for dealing with my knees as well as other aches and pains. You get a great sweat out of every class and always leave feeling refreshed. It's truly *hotness* (LOL)!

CHAPTER 15

"At first, they'll ask you why you're doing it.

Then, they'll ask you how you did it."

On this journey to improve your appearance and health, you may find that the people around you are not as supportive as you would hope. They may not blatantly hate on you or what you are trying to accomplish. But, they will give you some indirect pushback. They will question why you are only eating certain things, become annoyed when you decline their offer to go get drinks, and roll their eyes when you tell them you have to go to the gym.

"Why are you doing all this?"

"You're fine the way you are! You don't need to do all that!"

"What are you trying to prove?"

And the list can go on. I want to stress that I do not believe that hate is their motive. I believe it is more of a subconscious issue that they have with themselves. They may aspire to have similar goals as you. But, they lack either the courage to get started, the know-how to achieve their goal, or the will power to commit to it. In either of those instances, you should encourage them to buy this book (LOL)! But for real...

But stay on the course. Stay focused on the goals that you have set for yourself. Eventually, you will notice the question changing from people being perplexed and asking, "Why are you doing this," to them being amazed and asking, "HOW DID YOU DO IT," as if something magically happened. Take this drastic change in reaction as validation for the work you have done, and let it fuel your fire further. That's #WhatWinnersDo.

Don't kill yourself over your scale.

MUSCLE > FAT

No item has killed more workout commitments, plans, and confidence than a scale. A person will have all the drive in the world, work out five days a week, and even eat right. But, if they get on that scale and do not get good news…the tears shall floweth (LOL)! I speak from experience when I tell you that a scale reading can be completely deflating, have you convinced you are wasting your time, and all the work you have done has been for nothing. But while the number on the scale is real, it does not necessarily tell the whole story.

If you are working out, you are constantly using your body's muscles. This will cause your muscles to become more developed and grow. Your body will basically burn fat and grow muscle. When comparing the two, **muscle has a higher density and simply weighs more than fat**.

I trained someone for an entire month. She was on a strict diet and did some form of workout (weights or cardio) six days a week. At the end of the month, I put her on the scale. Amazingly, she had only lost about 5 pounds. This, as you can imagine, for her was very disheartening. She even began to curse me out for wasting her time for the last month. She was heated! But then, we took her measurements. We found that her waist had gone from a size 8-10 down to a size 6! Needless to say, she gave SK a heartfelt apology. I was like, "WHEW!"

So, do not let that scale number discourage your hard work. I suggest going by your body measurements or body fat percentage. There is a machine called a BOD POD™ where you can get a breakdown of your body mass. It will tell you how much of your total weight is bone, muscle, fat, water, and organs. This will allow you to see the progress of how much fat you have lost.

I got a test done, and my reading was 197 pounds with twelve percent body fat. This means that of my 197 pounds, roughly 24 pounds of that was fat. After six weeks of training, I went in for another reading and measured in at 200 pounds with ten percent body fat. While I actually gained three pounds during that time, I lost four pounds of fat and gained six pounds of muscle. That represented some very good progress.

Now, it may be a bit challenging to find a place with a BOD POD, where you can get measured. My friend, Dr. Michele Reid, the nationally known health coach, is who I personally go to. You will have to do a bit of research to find one in your area. People may tell you to just use a device called *the gun* to measure your body fat. It is used by taking a grab of three areas on your body and then giving you a number. I will tell you that this instrument is neither ideally accurate nor consistent. But, if it's the only tool you have available, use it, and keep those facts in mind.

side note for ladies Do not compare your progress with a man. A woman's body needs more fat than a man. Plus, women burn fat slower. So if you are working out with your husband or boyfriend, do not become depressed if his results are happening faster than yours!

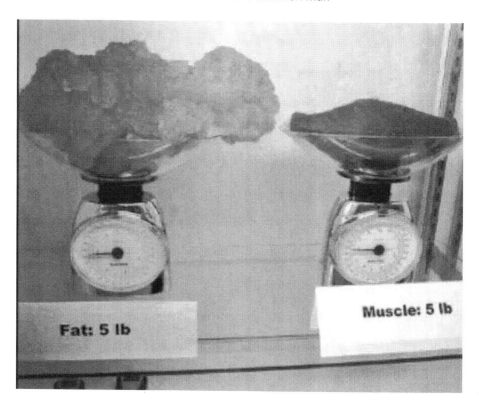

The illustration above shows five pounds of fat versus five pounds of muscle. As you can see,
the five pounds of fat takes up significantly more space than the five pounds of muscle. Also,
the five pounds of muscle is a lot smoother in texture, which looks much better when
pressed against your skin.

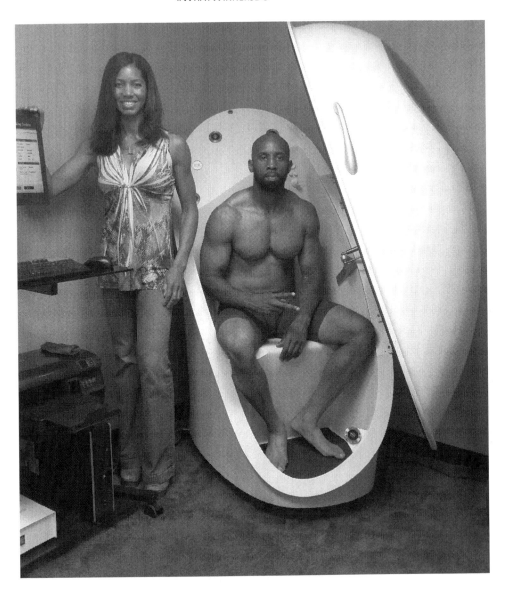

Michele, The Fitness Coach, is my go-to person to get my BOD POD reading. She is also helpful with great dieting and lifestyle tips.

CONCLUSION

People come to me a lot now, especially those who knew me before my transformation and ask some variation of the same questions:

"What's the best way?"

"How do I flourish on an epic level?"

That's not exactly what they say, but that's what they mean. My answer has two simple but major points: It takes a little know-how, and a lot of want-to.

Look, the things written in this book are things that I found that work for ME, SK, and for the most part, they are universally accepted as truths. But, every person's body is different. You have to experiment with different things in order to learn what works best for you. What works for SK may not exactly work for you and vice versa. A prime example is Willis, the Ab Technician, and I work out together often. Willis generally eats before every workout. His logical explanation that "you wouldn't drive your car without putting gas in it" is hard to argue. Meanwhile, if I eat before a workout, I feel sluggish and often vomit during the course of training. Therefore, I eat afterwards. On the other hand, I drink water constantly through the course of training, if for no other reason than to keep from getting the white mouth. Willis, on the other hand, drinks absolutely no water until he's done. This is just a simple example of how two people's bodies can be different.

Now, everyone you meet will swear to you that they have the answer! They will swear their way is best, and if you are not doing it their way, then you're losing. Just remember, every frog praises his own pond. **Whether its food, workouts, or lifestyle habits, NOBODY knows exactly what will work for YOU!** It's on you to use trial and error to figure out what works best. So train with other trainers, take random boot camps, accept invitations to work out with friends, and experiment with different types of exercise classes such as yoga, CrossFit, swimming, boxing, or Pilates. Do all these things until you develop the know-how that helps YOU flourish.

Now, for the want-to. By far, this is the most important and hardest thing to maintain on your quest. Two things I can promise you: It will not be easy, and it will not happen overnight. It takes days and days, weeks and weeks, months and months to achieve real change. So many people start off with a fire and determination to change their bodies, but turn cold and get discouraged along the way because they do not see immediate results.

There is a parable about a man determined to break a boulder. The story goes, he swung his pick axe, and hit the rock. But, nothing happened. So he swung again. Still nothing happened. He swung again, and again, and again. Still absolutely nothing happened. After the 501st swing, he looked. But still nothing happened. He continued swinging, with the same result, until on the 1000th swing, he struck the boulder and it split in half right down the middle. The man stood up, pleased with his work, and realized that it was not the 1000th hit that broke the boulder. It was the accumulation of ALL the previous swings that got the job done.

That parable displays the journey you will be on and the type of commitment you will need to get those great results you want. They will not come easy, and I can tell you from personal experience that it will take awhile before you will even notice. There will be many days that you look at yourself in the mirror and say, "I look the exact same...What the *hell* am I doing all this for?!" Discouragement will try to set in, and you may want to stop...BUT DON'T!! Keep swinging your pick axe! Keep going forward! Keep grinding hard! Keep pushing yourself! I promise you the results will come!

Look at me (pages 3, 16), I do not have a perfect body by any means. But I look *damn* good! I promise you it's not because of great genetics, any type of vanity surgeries, or any steroids or HGH. I got to where I am by staying determined and by seeking and using all the information and advice I could get along the way. Please do not get it twisted; it was *damn* hard to get here. Everything you have read in this book comes from my personal experience; from the workout advice, all the way to the self-doubting thoughts that could possibly go through your head. It always baffles me when someone says, "Man SK, I could never get my body to look that good (Insert confused Jackie Chan face)." Huh?! Why not?! There's nothing special about me. There's nothing to separate you and me to where you would say, "Well I don't have the ability to do what SK did." I'm not Kobe Bryant, I'm not Adrian Peterson, Channing Tatum, Terry Crews, or LeBron James. I'm a regular, everyday person JUST LIKE YOU! And just like SK, YOU CAN DO IT! You can have a six-pack stomach! You can have nice legs! You can have a firm butt! You can have a chiseled chest! You have the ability to transform your body into whatever you want it to look like. All that's stopping you is you.

How can I be so sure? Because I see how you flourish in other aspects of your life. Whether it's your career, taking care of your home, or raising your children, you do truly amazing things in your life that are greater than or equal to what it would take to transform your body. A friend of mine told me that she couldn't get a flat stomach because it was too hard. The crazy thing is that she's a doctor! I watched her go through years of medical school, which consisted of constant fifteen-hour study days, AND NOW YOU"RE TELLING ME YOU CANNOT MUSTER UP THE STRENGTH TO DISCPLINE YOUR DIET AND WORKOUT HABITS?! (My high-pitched Atlanta voice) REALLY SHAWTY?! It does not add up. The reality is that you, like her, do indeed have the ability to change yourself. But you lack the will and confidence to push yourself to exceed your limits. Somewhere along the way, you were made to believe it is not realistic for you to flourish on that level. Do not believe that lie! Unlearn that hogwash! Attack this challenge with the same vigor that you use for anything else you deem important in your life. That's the way you will get it to happen for you.

So figure out what you want to look like, set up workouts, change your diet, ask questions from everyone you know, give it your best day in and day out, and if you stay the course long enough, I promise you will flourish and reach your goals. Then on that day, you will look at yourself in the mirror, with a huge smirk on your face, and you'll say ever so proudly, "NOW THAT'S WHAT WINNERS DO!"

#WhatWinnersDo

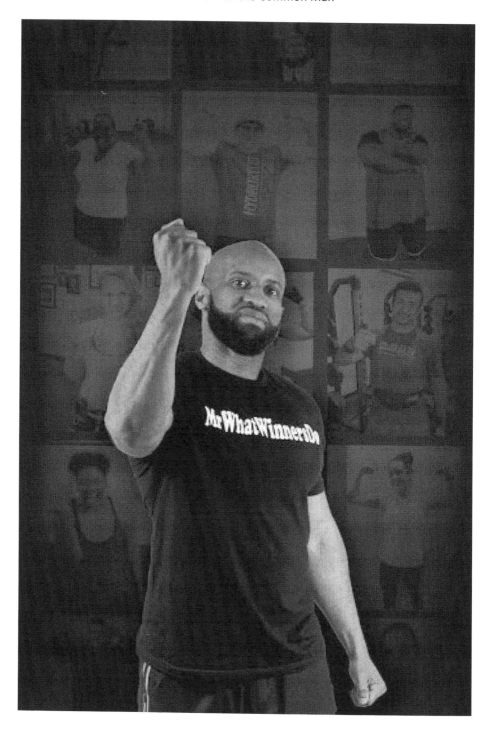

#WhatWinnersDo

REVIEW

EXERCISING

- Work out consistently for better physical appearance and health.
- SQUATS! Learn them, and do them often.
- Plank to work your abs effectively.
- Speed up your workouts to burn more calories and fat.
- Change your workout routines to keep your body from plateauing.
- Cardio. I know you hate it, but you got to get it in.
- Push through pain and discomfort. BUT understand, if you think you're injured, STOP IMMEDIATELY!!

DIETING

- Stay away from the white stuff!
- Eat as clean as possible, as often as possible.
- Eat your meals the same time everyday.
- Stay away from eating late at night.
- Avoid buffets, fast food, and high-fructose corn syrup.
- Drink water first thing when you wake up, before every meal, and before you go to bed.

MISCELLANEOUS

- Sleep the same amount at the same time daily.
- Remember muscle has more density than fat. So pay more attention to changes in size than scale numbers.

#WhatWinnersDo

NOTES

SK's Fitness Plan for the Common Man

#WhatWinnersDo

SK's Fitness Plan for the Common Man

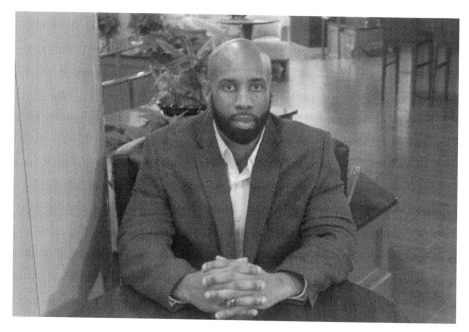

Steven SK Kennedy received his bachelors of science in Electrical Engineering from the University of South Carolina. A true student-athlete, SK overcame the difficulties of being an engineer major and a varsity football player. As a devoted trainee, Steven has trained under the tutelage of University of Texas head strength coach Pat Moore, world record holder Dan Austin, collegiate strength coach Mark Smith, fitness professional Ken Taylor, and body building trainers Larry Lockhart and Jack Barron. Intense training under their mentorship has given SK the breadth of Knowledge to create a program for the common everyday person. SK currently works full-time as a benefits specialist for Colonial Life. He is also a motivational speaker, fitness consultant, and is a football coach in Columbia, SC.

First, I would like to thank Jesus Christ, my Lord and Savior. At my lowest moment, I prayed to you and confessed, "I've gotten myself into a situation, and the only chance I have of getting out is through you." You delivered me from that place and never abandoned me. I know that whatever success I achieve and whatever heights I reach are not because of my own doing but because of your grace and mercy. I will forever sing your praise and give you the glory.

I would like to thank my parents for everything they have done. Through all the mistakes and bad decisions I've made, the both of you stayed patient with me. You continuously gave me your unwavering support and unconditional love. I love the two of you more than I could possibly articulate. Thank you to both of my grandmothers. The both of you have meant so much in shaping my spiritual beliefs and work habits. I feel your prayers from above and beyond the grave. Granddad Spooky, I will never forget you or the bond we shared. I miss you and will love you forever. Cuz, thank you for being the great person you are. Watching you constantly achieve and conquer new goals has always been truly inspiring to me. Your consistent support and positive energy have meant so much to my growth and this book.

My boys, Dan the Man and Black Iron, I thank the both of you so much for looking out for me. Y'all took me under your wings, treated me like a little brother, and really set the foundation for my fitness transformation by showing me how to really work (#salute). Coach Holtz, I am still in awe of the amount of wisdom that I was able to gain from you over those years. Playing under your leadership was truly a pleasure.

Ryan and Keith, thanks for helping me conquer new heights (LOL)! Bang Gang bro!! Ken, thanks for dropping those nuggets of great information every morning and for always being supportive. Ham, I appreciate the time and effort you always put into coming up with new ideas for me to get better. I'll always support you. Jack, Roc, Eazy, and Mohawk, thanks for putting me on with y'all and showing me another level. Steel Mill Fam Forever.

SK's Fitness Plan for the Common Man

To my boy Will, this doesn't happen on this level without you. Thanks for getting my vision out of my head and making it a reality. Brandy, thank you for turning this into a quality production. I appreciate your willingness to fight with me through my stubbornness in order to make this happen. Ty, thanks for being the jerk lawyer I needed you to be. Tesha, buddy, you saved SK multiple times. Thanks for being my personal tech support! Sunshine, thank you for coaching me up and slowing me down. PT, I really appreciate all the sit downs we had and jewels we shared. BB, thank you for all your helpful suggestions. You came through in the clutch, like the star you are!

To all my family, friends, and supporters, y'all are everything to me. The encouraging words, optimistic support, constructive criticism, and silly jokes give me life on a daily bases. PBP, GC, Sports Zone, Lion's Den, FB Fam, E, Bgood, BC, Ross, Sugar, JG, Redan, Eastside, Conway, Metro, Myrtle Beach, and everybody in between, I love y'all from the bottom of my heart.

Sincerely your favorite homie,

SK, Mr. WhatWinnersDo